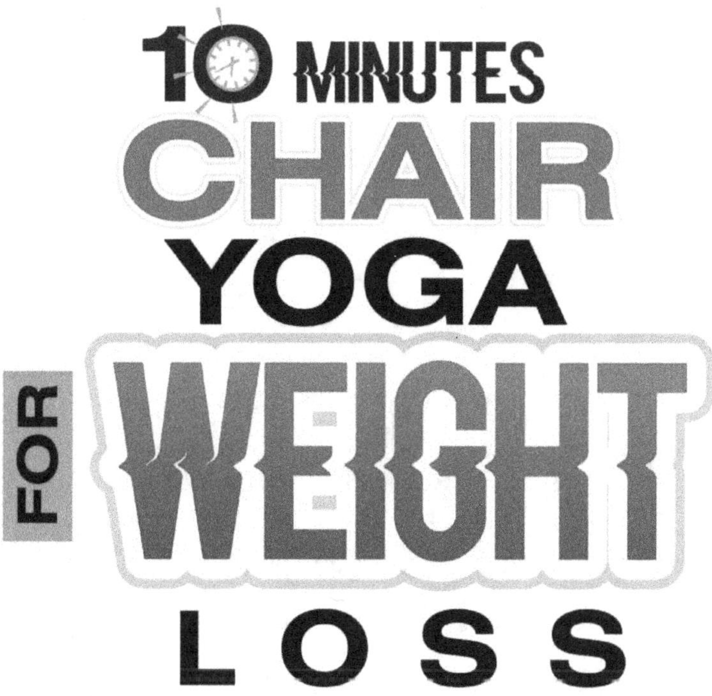

10 MINUTES CHAIR YOGA FOR WEIGHT LOSS

Gentle Exercises for Seniors and Beginners: Quick and Easy Home Workouts with Proven Delicacies

DR. JESSICA REEVES

TABLE OF CONTENT

Introduction

EXPLORING THE WORKS OF CHAIR YOGA

This moderate style of yoga is known as chair yoga, and it is performed while seated on a chair or with the assistance of a chair's support. It is a modified form of conventional yoga that makes the practice accessible to anyone who may have trouble practicing yoga on a mat, such as senior citizens, individuals with mobility challenges, or those who have worries about their balance.

For chair yoga, practitioners execute yoga postures and exercises while seated or utilizing a chair for support. This makes it much simpler to keep one's balance and stability under control. Flexibility, strength, and relaxation are all areas that may be improved via the practice of chair yoga, which can involve relaxing stretching, breathing exercises, and meditation techniques. The practice of chair yoga may be useful for people of all ages and fitness levels. Still, it can be beneficial for people who have physical restrictions or ailments that make traditional yoga difficult to do. Improvements in posture, stress reduction, increased flexibility, and general well-being are all possible outcomes of this practice.

Chair yoga courses are offered in a variety of locations, including community centers, yoga studios, and senior centers. Additionally, there are online resources and videos accessible for anyone who would rather carry out their practice at home. It is a good idea to contact a healthcare physician or a competent yoga instructor if you are interested in attempting chair yoga. This will guarantee that the practice is safe and suitable for your specific requirements on an individual level.

Chair Yoga's Many Benefits for Weight Loss Comprises

In today's fast-paced environment, keeping a healthy weight is vital for general well-being. While traditional forms of exercise may not be accessible to everyone, chair yoga offers a gentle yet effective technique to promote weight reduction and improve fitness. Chair yoga is a comfortable alternative for persons with restricted mobility, physical restraints, or those who are just starting their fitness journey. This article investigates how chair yoga may be a beneficial tool for weight management and includes some successful positions to get you started.

The Benefits of Chair Yoga for Weight Loss:

1. Low Impact: Chair yoga is a low-impact type of exercise, making it suited for people of all fitness levels. It lowers

pressure on joints while yet helping burn calories and enhance cardiovascular health.

2. Muscle Engagement: Chair yoga postures activate numerous muscle groups, helping to strengthen and tone muscles. As muscles expand, they boost your basal metabolic rate, resulting in more calories expended even at rest.

3. Stress Reduction: Stress and emotional problems might lead to weight gain. Chair yoga involves deep breathing and relaxation methods that can decrease stress, lower cortisol levels, and encourage mindful eating habits.

4. Improved Digestion: Certain chair yoga positions can stimulate the digestive tract, assisting in digestion and minimizing bloating. This can help to a healthy gut and simpler weight reduction journey.

5. Increased Flexibility: As you practice chair yoga frequently, your flexibility and range of motion will increase. This can lead to better posture and body alignment, increasing overall confidence and body image.

Effective Chair Yoga Poses for Weight Loss:

1. Seated Spinal Twist: This position helps accelerate digestion, increase spinal flexibility, and activate core muscles.

2. Chair Cat-Cow: Similar to the conventional cat-cow stance, this sitting form maintains a healthy spine and works abdominal muscles.

3. Seated Forward Fold: This position stretches the hamstrings, lower back, and shoulders, enhancing flexibility and lowering stress.

4. Chair Warrior II: Engage your leg muscles and extend your hips with this position, boosting lower body strength and balance.

5. Seated Sun Salutation: A modified variation of the original sun salutation, this sequence warms up the body, improves circulation, and raises energy levels.

Incorporating Chair Yoga into Your Routine:

1. Consistency: Aim for a regular chair yoga practice, gradually increasing the time and intensity as your fitness improves.

2. Breath Awareness: Focus on deep and thoughtful breathing during each position. This not only boosts the efficiency of the workouts but also helps control stress.

3. Listen to Your Body: Chair yoga should never cause discomfort. If a position is painful, alter it or omit it completely.

4. Seek Guidance: Join a chair yoga class or watch online instructions to verify you're doing postures correctly and securely.

Conclusion: Chair yoga is a fantastic alternative for people seeking a mild yet impactful fitness regimen for weight loss. By activating muscles, lowering tension, improving flexibility, and aiding digestion, chair yoga offers a comprehensive approach to reaching and maintaining a healthy weight. Remember that any weight reduction journey requires time and consistency, so be patient with yourself and enjoy the process of improving your entire well-being with chair yoga.

How to get started with Chair Yoga

Chair yoga is one of the safest methods to practice yoga and is the best sort of yoga for anyone who has mobility concerns, is just starting, has had a recent injury, or would prefer extra assistance when trying advanced postures. When compared to other types of yoga, it's considerably kinder on your limbs since you have the support of the chair anytime you need it.

What to look for in Yoga chair

Whether you are performing standing yoga or inversions, a comfortable chair will provide you with the support you require. Before you purchase a yoga chair, you need to know what characteristics to search for and what to consider, as there are many various types of yoga chairs on the market. Think about:

A yoga chair should be comfy.

The right yoga chair has to be comfy for you. It should give the support you need to complete tough yoga postures and shouldn't be too bulky. Look for a chair that has soft material so it doesn't push against your skin or get slippery when you start to sweat.

A yoga chair should be lightweight and easy to transport.

The yoga chair you purchase should be light and simple to carry about. You shouldn't be bound to practicing in one spot, so having a hefty chair that isn't movable might become a headache. If you intend on taking a yoga class or traveling on yoga retreats, you'll want a chair that you can easily carry with you.

Why can't I just use a normal chair for chair yoga?

The benefit of utilizing a yoga chair is that it was created and developed for yoga. A conventional chair, while it might be more handy, wasn't meant to work on or, for that matter, sweat on. An excellent yoga chair will be manufactured from a non-slip material that's easy to clean and that can bear a certain amount of weight (particularly if you'll be performing inversions). All in all, utilizing a yoga chair helps lower your risk of being harmed.

Top 7 Chairs Yoga: The finest yoga chairs

Aozora Backless Yoga Chair Prop

The Aozora backless yoga chair provides you extra support wherever you practice yoga, while still providing you adequate freedom to walk around thanks to the wide-open back. It's also double-hinged, making it highly strong so you can feel secure performing any sort of position.

Tonchean Yoga Chair with Back Support

This yoga chair is low in weight — making it easy to move from one spot to another or take about with you. Not only is the linen fabric non-slip, it's also dirt-resistant and breathable. This yoga chair also comes with retractable waist support and has hooved feet so it won't slide around on your yoga mat (or the ground).

CIGOCIVI Yoga Support Chair with Lumbar Backrest

This yoga chair is a terrific alternative for a broad range of yoga postures as it supports your back and hip movement. It comes with lumbar support, which is also detachable. The frame is composed of aluminum while the cushions are made from sponge. You can fold it up and put it away when you're not using it, and it comes with a 1-year warranty that promises to replace the chair if it breaks or wears.

Pune Yoga Chair

This is a simple, backless folding chair that's excellent if you're searching for a basic chair to support you during your yoga courses. It's lightweight, collapsible, and robust enough that you can lean into it.

The finest yoga inversion chairs

KOKSRY Yoga Headstand Bench, Foldable Yoga Inversion Chair: available at Amazon

Inversion yoga postures are an integral aspect of any advanced yoga regimen. Therefore, having a yoga chair that supports you as you do inversions is crucial. The KOKSRY Yoga Chair is a high-quality device with a firm PU cushion meant to remove any stress from your neck. This cushion gives the optimum support for your head, neck, and shoulders.

Puluomis Yoga Headstand Bench

This yoga chair has a superb ergonomic design that assists with all your inversion needs. It gives ideal support for your neck and shoulders, keeping you safe in advanced postures without worrying about generating strain on your head and neck. It's built from birch wood and plush faux leather cushioning. There are two components to this chair: you can use it together like a cushioned stool or remove one of the portions, leaving a U-shaped cushion that's perfect for going upside down.

SISYAMA Inversion Bench Yoga Headstand Chair

This is another inversion chair that's excellent for anyone looking to enhance their upside-down flexibility safely. Unlike other inversion chairs, it comes with a broader and thicker cushion and comes with an instructional booklet so you can immediately learn how to use it properly. This design also contains self-locking hooks to aid in keeping it in place.

Chapter 1

THE FUNDAMENTALS OF CHAIR YOGA

Basic Chair Yoga Poses

Most chair yoga poses need you to sit forward on the seat—away from the back of the chair—so that you can move more freely. But the chair back may also work as a prop to provide you greater support and leverage, especially in twisting poses. As in any yoga session, you may also wish to keep blocks or a strap (or belt) available when doing chair yoga postures to help you in finding a version that works for you.

1. Upward Salute Pose (Urdhva Hastasana)

Upward Salute is a terrific method to extend your arms and shoulders while stretching your spine.

1. Sit with your back a few inches from the back of the chair. Lengthen your spine, stretching the crown of your head up and softly releasing your tailbone toward the seat. Raise your chin so it is parallel to the ground.

2. Place your feet flat on the floor with your big toes touching and a little space between your heels. (If you have lower back pain, practice with your feet hip-distance apart. Place

your feet on blocks if they don't reach the floor.) Root down with your big toe mounds, your heels, and the outer edges of your feet.

3. Inhale, bring your shoulders back, relax your front ribs, and lift your arms aloft with your hands shoulder-distance apart and palms facing each other. If your shoulders are tense, take your arms broader than your shoulders.

4. Reach your fingers toward the ceiling and keep your eyes straight ahead. If you like, you can touch your hands together and bring your sight to your thumbs.

5. Keep your arms strong. Stay here for many breaths. Release your arms.

2. Cat Pose (Marjaryasana)

As in the more recognized variant of Cat Pose practiced from hands and knees, you want to simultaneously circle your back as you pull your chin into your chest. This helps enhance flexibility in the spine and extends the shoulders.

1. Sit on the chair with your feet hip-width apart.
2. Rest your hands on your knees.
3. On an exhale, curve your spine and lower your chin into your chest.
4. Take many comfortable breaths here. On an exhale, slowly roll your head up and return to the previous posture.

5. Dark-haired woman with rust-colored tights and top practices Cow Pose in a chair

3. Cow Pose (Bitilasana)

You might recall Cow Pose from the back-to-back sequence of Cat Pose and Cow Pose that is commonly cued on all fours in a yoga class. This seated variant is still a backbend in which you elevate your chest and your eyes. Similar to Cat Pose, it can help you build flexibility in the spine.

1. Sit on the chair with your feet and knees hip-width apart. Let your hands rest on your thighs or knees.
2. Inhale and arch your back. Lengthen around the back of your neck and your lower back to produce a long, uniform curvature.
3. Lift your chin and sternum, expand your collarbones, and allow your shoulders to fall back and away from your ears.
4. Take several breaths. Slowly drop your chin and return to a neutral spine.

4. Camel Pose (Ustrasana)

You'll feel stretching and strengthening of the chest, upper back, and shoulders in this sitting form of Camel Pose.

1. Sit on the chair with your feet hip-width apart.

2. Inhale and arch your upper back, letting your shoulder blades contact the back of your chair. (It's alright if your shoulders do not contact the back of the chair; merely focus on arching your back and elevating your eyes without straining.)

3. Lift your chin and sternum, expand your collarbones, and allow your shoulders to fall back and away from your ears.

4. If it's comfortable, extend your arms back to hold the legs of the chair. Rotate your arms externally so that the inside of your elbows face front.

5. On your next inhalation, elevate your chest, enabling your rib cage to expand and generating a long, even curve through your mid and upper back. You may push your feet onto the floor to work your legs and core.

6. Take several breaths. To exit the pose, release your hands, tuck your chin, and return to your original sitting position.

5. Happy Baby Pose (Ananda Balasana)

In this sitting form of Happy Baby, you can keep your spine straight or allow your back and shoulders to circle forward while you relax your neck.

1. Sit near the front edge of the chair with your feet on the floor, a bit wider than hip-width apart.

2. Reach the crown of your head up and drag your tailbone down to discover the length of your back.

3. As you exhale, bend forward at your hips and pull your tummy between your thighs. You may opt to expand your legs to generate extra room for your body.

4. Inhale and reach down between your thighs and grip your outside shins, ankles, or feet.

5. Gently draw your torso down between your thighs, lowering your body toward the floor.

6. Take several breaths. To release the posture, let go of your grasp and activate your core muscles as you lift your head, neck, shoulders, and torso to return to your original sitting position.

6. King Arthur's Pose

In King Arthur's Pose, you may adjust the stretch in your quadriceps by shifting the location of your ankle. Bring your ankle closer to your hip for a more severe stretch, or farther away for a softer stretch.

1. Sit in a chair with your sit bones in the middle of the seat. Shift your weight to the right side of the seat and position your feet level on the floor with your knees hip-width apart.

2. Keep your right leg attached to the chair seat as you bend your right knee, lift your foot off the floor, and point your toes toward the back of the chair.

3. Reach down with your right hand and hold your ankle. Gently push it toward your body until you feel a powerful stretch in your quadricep and the front of your shin. (If you can't reach your ankle, thread a strap or cloth over your foot.)

4. Take several breaths. Lower your foot and return to your previous sitting posture. Repeat on the opposite side.

7. Tree Pose (Vrksasana)

Tree position is meant as a stretch for the hips, a strengthening of the hamstrings, as well as a balancing position. It gives everything of the aforementioned in the sitting variant.

1. Sit nearer the front edge of the chair. Inhale deeply, elevate your chest and exhale as you bring your shoulder blades down your back. Look straight ahead at a steady gazing position.

2. Extend your left leg straight out in front of you. Position your foot by either flexing it or pointing your toes toward the floor.

3. Open your right leg out to the side, keeping your knee bent and your foot or toes on the floor.

4. Place your hands in anjali mudra, or prayer position, at your heart or stretch your arms upwards.

5. Take several breaths. To release the posture, plant your right leg back into the seat, and land both feet firmly on the floor. Come back to your previous sitting posture. Mirror the position on the opposite side.

8. Extended Triangle Pose (Utthita Trikonasana)

Extended Triangle Pose stretches the thighs, hips, lower back, and torso, which makes it a perfect stretch for muscles that are tight from extended sitting. Listen to your body and turn your attention anyplace that feels most comfortable, whether straight ahead, at your elevated arm, or down at your leg.

1. Sit such that your torso is on the left side of the chair and your left leg clears the seat.

2. Stretch your left leg straight out to the side. Firm your thigh and straighten your leg as much as possible.

3. Inhale and raise your arms straight out from your shoulders and parallel to the floor. Keep your shoulder blades broad and your palms down.

4. Exhale and tilt your torso to the left, bending from your hip joint. Reach your left arm out and down toward your outstretched leg, putting your left hand on your shin or thigh. Extend your right arm upward toward the ceiling.

5. Keep your head in a neutral position or turn to look either at your right hand or down at the floor.

6. Take several breaths. Inhale and come back to sitting. Shift your body to the right side of your chair and repeat the stance on the opposite side.

9. Bound Angle Pose (Baddha Konasana)

Taking your feet farther away from you in Bound Angle Pose offers a less intense stretch if having your feet closer to the chair seems too strenuous. Don't force the stretch.

1. Sit near the front edge of the chair so that your buttocks are supported but your knees clear the seat.

2. Open your legs wide, such that your knees point away from each other.

3. Sit tall, pushing your shoulder blades on your upper back to raise through your sternum. Extend the top of your head upward toward the ceiling.

4. Keep your knees wide as you bring your feet together. Open your feet as if you were opening the pages of a book, keeping the outside borders of your feet together.

5. Place your hands on your thighs and gently push your thighs away from each other.

6. Take several breaths. Slowly disengage and return to your initial sitting posture.

10. High Lunge

This sitting-high lunge stretches your thigh muscles and strengthens your hips, knees, and ankles.

1. Sit on your chair facing the left side of the room so that your thighs are fully supported. Shift toward the front of the chair so that your right leg clears the seat.
2. Keeping both hips looking front, stretch your right leg straight back. Place the ball of your foot on the floor. Engage your right thigh by pulling it up toward the ceiling to straighten your leg as much as possible. Ensure that your left knee is aligned directly above your right ankle.
3. Inhale and stretch your arms toward the ceiling, keeping your shoulders open and your arms aligned with your ears.
4. Take several breaths. To exit the stance, release your arms and bring your right leg forward.
5. Shift in the seat to face the right side of the room and repeat the position on the other side.

11. Extended Side Angle Pose (Utthita Parsvakonasana)

Extended Side Angle Pose extends your extended leg while expanding your shoulders, chest, and hips. If it's not comfortable, your lower hand doesn't need to be on the floor. Use a block or any item you have at home to bring the floor to your hand instead. You'll still benefit from a side stretch.

1. Sit facing the left side of your chair so that your thighs are fully supported on the seat. Shift yourself to the right, at the front side of the chair, so that your right leg clears the seat.

2. Extend your right leg back. Turn your hips towards the front of the chair. Straighten your right leg and place the bottom of your right foot on the floor with your toes pointing forward.

3. Lean your body toward your left knee, hinging from your hips to bring your left arm toward the floor. Place your left fingers on the ground or a block, so your arm and shin are parallel.

4. Reach your right arm toward the ceiling. Extend it beside your right ear, palm facing the floor, or bend your right elbow and reach back to grip the back of the chair.

5. Rotate your torso to move your chest toward your upper arm. Turn your head to look toward the ceiling or maintain your gaze ahead if more comfortable.

6. Take several breaths. To release the pose, press yourself up with your left hand and pull your right leg in to return to your sitting position.

7. Turn on the chair to face the right side of the room and repeat the position on the other side.

12. Half Lord of the Fishes (Ardha Matsyendrasana)

Half Lord of the Fishes stretches your outer thighs and hips while stretching your spine. Don't employ force here. Rotate gently until you sense a stretch, then hold for a few breaths. Position yourself on the edge of your chair to ensure full support from the seat.

1. Cross your right leg over your left leg.
2. Inhale as you stretch your spine and elevate both arms toward the ceiling.
3. Exhale and twist to the right as you bring your hands down to hold the back of the chair.
4. Turn your head to the right, peering past your right shoulder. Ensure you avoid putting undue strain on your neck.
5. Take several breaths. To release the posture, inhale and extend your arms up, and then exhale and unwind your body. Place both feet on the floor.
6. Turn to the left side of your chair and repeat the position on that side.

13. Marichyasana III

In sitting Marichyasana III, the twisting action gives for a stretch in your shoulders, hips, and lower back.

1. Sit with your spine supported by the back of the chair. Lengthen your spine and gradually relax your tailbone toward the seat.

2. Position your feet on the floor with a hip-width distance between them.

3. Lift your right knee and pull it toward your chest. Place your right foot on the seat of the chair as near to your right sitting bone as feasible.

4. Inhale and stretch your spine. Exhale and twist to the right. Hold your right knee with your left hand or encircle your right knee with your left elbow.

5. Drape your right arm over the back of the chair and either grab the chair back or clasp your hands together.

6. Take several breaths. Lengthen on each inhalation and gradually twist a bit more with each expiration.

7. To release the posture, drop your arms, unwind your body, and plant your right foot back on the floor. Repeat on the opposite side.

Safety Tips and Modifications for chair yoga

First and foremost: Yoga is not about the positions, it's about the breath. It's about the breath linking the mind, body, and spirit so that you may access the proven benefits that the breath and the asanas (poses) bring throughout the body. It's about the breath helping you control your thoughts versus your thoughts dominating you. It's about learning to calm your thoughts. Yoga is a movement meditation under the guidance of the breath.

Yoga is not a competitive sport, it's a personal practice. NEVER compete with the individuals next to you or the teacher. And never be scared or ashamed to employ physical adjustments or items like blocks and straps. Yoga is also a non-judgmental practice. If you can't quite touch the floor and I can touch my hands to the floor, you should utilize blocks or go to your shins. We are both getting the same advantage. If you hang out instead of asking the teacher for blocks or utilizing your shins, you are setting yourself up to damage your lower back, and not stand out because you are the only person using blocks. And while it is nice to want to push yourself, it's not going too deep into a posture that gets you to your objective you are more likely to damage yourself. You MUST LISTEN TO YOUR BODY. Just because you could effortlessly glide into a pigeon position yesterday, doesn't imply your body will comply today. The key to attaining new milestones in strength, flexibility, meditation, and balance is to maintain regular practice.

If you wish to practice just under the supervision of a DVD or YouTube personality, go to a studio and attend a few lessons under a teacher who can help you understand the right procedural and safety concerns, and the proper breathing methods so you stay healthy and safe throughout your home practice.

While this is by NO means a comprehensive list, here are a few safety precautions.

Asana Safety:

1. To aid with the protection of your back and appropriate development of your core, draw your belly button toward your spine during and transitioning between asanas. Don't "suck in" and hold your breath. Instead, envision a thread tied to the rear of the belly button and coming out of your back. Imagine tugging the string so the belly button pushes back and slightly up. (To assist in illustrating the following point, this drawing of the belly is one of the bandha locks called Uddiyana Bandha) KEEP BREATHING!

2. Because many of my students, as well as myself, have lower back problems, I also advocate activating the Mula Bandha (PLEASE Google this phrase, as it is more comprehensive than I can describe in words.) I hate to put it this basic without additional teaching, however, I have many students who walk in with back problems new to a class and need to know a method to reach the activation without a lengthy anatomy course. I tell ladies it is like drawing in with the biggest kegel available to them. When

they add it to #1, they lock together and protect the back. For guys, I tell them to pretend like they are halting their urinating midstream.

3. When standing in postures that involve bending your front leg(s), like in Warrior I, your knee should always be above the heel. Never allow your knees to bend past your toes. You should be able to see at LEAST your first two toes if not all of them. When practicing Warriors I and II, triangle, pyramid, side angle, etc remember to line up the front heel with either the rear heel or the arch of the back foot. In the standing stance chair, where both knees are bent you should place the weight on the heels and be able to wriggle your toes. (Wiggling your toes is not part of the posture, it merely enables you to make sure you are standing properly.) Again, you should be able to see your toes.

4. Headstands, shoulder stands, plows, etc. NEVER try anything that includes the neck without a qualified teacher working with you and spotting you. In terms of headstands, many teachers no longer incorporate headstands in their practice since they CAN be harmful. If you roll your neck, or it isn't stable before you elevate your legs, you may compress discs, and strain muscles, and though I've never seen it, you could break your neck. I make sure a thick pad is under the head and I make sure that the learner enters

into a tripod stand to measure the strength of their neck. I adore headstands, but I have been doing them my whole life. Recently I got a headstand stool that allows you to execute a headstand without your head ever hitting the floor. In terms of shoulder stands, plow stance, or similar, your neck should NEVER contact the floor. Your teacher should be able to place his/her hand under your neck to verify there is a gap between your neck and the floor.

5. Be conscious of your transitions. It's quite simple to get caught up in BEING in the next posture, that we don't pay attention to getting there. A high number of injuries occur during the transition between positions. All movements should be purposefully and thoughtfully done.

6. Never lock your arms or knees.

7. Don't overdo the Chaturanga. Yes, they are nice and create strength in your arms and your core. But doing too many will hurt your shoulders.

8. Every action has an opposing action or response. If you twist one direction, twist the other. If you bend your spine one way, bend it the other. Mirror the movement on both sides, similar to the cat/cow pose in yoga.

Chapter 2

DAILY 10-MINUTE CHAIR YOGA ROUTINES

Morning Energizer Routine

My morning routine owes itself to my night routine. That is, I feel that less is more when it comes to the morning.

Why?

Because night rituals are only limited by the time you want to be sleeping. Morning routines are constrained by bus timetables, meetings, and traffic jams - factors that are not in your control.

 For example, here are the things I get ready before going to bed:

- I choose my clothing and lunch for the next day.
- I decide on my breakfast.
- I shower
- I determine what bus I need to take to work and what bus I will take if I miss that one.

I do things so that I don't even need to think about them in the morning.

Simplicity is crucial to decreasing morning anxiety.

And so long as my morning anxiety is minimal, my day is likely to be quite nice.

The other component of achieving simplicity in your routines is recognizing the things that are significant for you. Not for everyone.

For example, I have a SAD light treatment lamp that I sit next to for around 20 minutes in the morning. Would I suggest this to everyone?

Maybe everyone in Northern latitudes, where it becomes quite dark in the winter. But this isn't going to be impactful for everyone. I found out that this light considerably enhances my motivation and energy by simply testing it.

I also got a really serious worry from infancy that I constantly need to be getting enough exercise. If I go for a 20-minute run in the morning, that paranoia is quiet.

Should everyone consider going for a run in the morning? Not necessarily. Some individuals might find it more stressful to integrate something into their schedule, prompting them to rush.

If anything is going to worsen your morning anxiety, then you probably shouldn't do it.

Simply said, the net benefit of adding something to your routine ought to be positive.

Yeah, jogging makes me more exhausted, but it also silences that paranoia, which is worth far more energy.

In summary, my preferred morning routine involves getting out of bed and spending 20 minutes next to my SAD lamp, accompanied by a light snack such as a banana while I think about the day ahead (sometimes taking notes in Evernote), go for a 20-minute run, take a quick shower just to rinse off the sweat, dress in my pre-selected clothes, eat my pre-selected breakfast, and head out for my pre-selected bus with my pre-selected lunch.

To me, that is the ultimate anxiety-quenching routine.

I don't believe in getting up 3 hours before you need to come to work to write creatively or prepare a smoothie from veggies in your garden.

Maybe that's because I'm not a real morning person. But what I do know is that I want to get up without feeling like I have a pile of things to accomplish.

Midday Stretch and Strengthen

As a working professional, it's easy to feel the consequences of sitting at a desk for hours on end. From neck and shoulder pain to back discomfort and hip stiffness, the toll of a sedentary lifestyle may be felt throughout the body.

What's the solution? Plan basic stretches to undertake during your mid-day break.

Incorporating stretches into your daily work routine will help you avoid the negative effects and even prevent more significant joint health concerns down the line and also you will enjoy benefits such as:

- The better mood at work
- Higher energy and alertness
- Refocus your mind
- Relax your body Improve your overall well-being
- Improve flexibility and mobility in joints
- Reduce stiffness in muscles

Easy Stretching Exercises for Home and Office Settings:

1. Overhead Stretch

This exercise focuses on the upper body, notably the shoulders and arms, developing flexibility and reducing stress in the neck and shoulders. It helps improve posture, reduce stiffness, and expand the range of motion in the upper body.

How to Perform the Overhead Stretch?

- Inhale, Raise your arms over your head, and push towards the ceiling.
- Exhale, Bring the hands to the chest.
- Keep your arms straight.

2. Neck Rolls

Neck discomfort is a typical concern for many people who work at desks, as they often strain their necks. This stretch helps release tension in the sides and back of your neck, decreasing discomfort and enhancing flexibility.

How to Perform Neck Rotation Exercise?

- Gently spin your head anticlockwise.
- Slowly pull your head back to the center.
- Now, slowly rotate your head in the other direction.
- Repeat this 3-4 times.

3. Side Bend Stretch

The Side Bend Stretch is a pleasant method to reduce stiffness and promote flexibility. By gradually extending the muscles along your side body, this stretch produces a sensation of release and renewal, allowing you to move with more ease and comfort.

How to Perform the Side Bend Stretch?

- Raise your arms over your head.
- Slowly bend your body to the left and then to the right.
- Repeat this exercise a few times.

4. Seated Pigeon Pose

This exercise targets the muscles in the glutes and hips, widely used to ease lower back pain by relieving tension in these muscle groups. It also helps to ease stiff hips, reduce tiredness, and improve posture.

How to Perform a Seated Pigeon Pose?

Cross one leg over the other while sitting, producing a figure four [i.e 4]

- Lean forward gradually from the hips, stretching fingertips towards the floor.
- Keep your arms straight.
- You should feel the strain in your buttocks.
- Hold the posture for a few moments.

5. Spinal Twists

Spinal twists stretch your spine, strengthen your back and abdominal muscles, enhance spinal flexibility, and help alleviate back discomfort.

How to Perform Spinal Twists?

- Extend your arms in front and slowly twist from the waist to the right.
- Breathe in, and return to the center.
- Breathe out, then repeat the same on your left side.
- Repeat this a few times.

6. Arm Rotation

Doing this activity frequently might help you relax your body and feel less worried and nervous, especially because we tend to sit stationary a lot.

How to Perform Arm Rotation Correctly?

- With feet shoulder-width apart, start circling your arms
- Next, do the same in the other way
- Repeat this a couple more times

7. Chest Extension

This workout targets the muscles in the shoulders and chest. The chest muscles support the shoulder joints, promote mobility, and lessen the possibility of shoulder injuries while simultaneously strengthening the upper body.

How to Perform Chest Extension Correctly?

- Extend the arms forward until they reach shoulder height, then bend the elbows.
- Bring the forearms together.
- Stretch the chest muscles.

Evening Relaxation Sequence

A Quick 10-Minute Bedtime Yoga Routine for Relaxation and Better Sleep.

In this nighttime yoga practice, you'll take yourself through some peaceful forward bends and hip-openers. Allow yourself to calm down and connect to your body and your breath. By the end of the exercise, you'll feel the release of bodily and mental stress, leaving you better ready to fall asleep.

1. Child's Pose (Balasana)

Come onto your mat on your hands and knees. Separate your knees wide and pull your big toes together. Bring your hips toward your heels and lay your forehead on a block, folded blanket, or on the mat. Walk your hands forward and lay your forearms on the mat. Close your eyes. Allow yourself to feel the feelings in your body as you relax into a Child's Pose. Stay here for 5-10 deep breaths.

2. Cat-Cow (Marjaryasana Bitilasana)

Come back to your hands and knees with your wrists behind your shoulders and your knees beneath your hips. On an inhalation, slowly release your belly toward the floor and move your chest forward, generating a minor backbend in Cow Pose.

On your exhale, curve your back toward the ceiling in Cat Pose.

Sync your movement with your breath and go gently through these shapes at least 5 more times.

3. Downward-Facing Dog Pose (Adho Mukha Svanasana)

Start on hands and knees, then move your hands forward until your wrists align with where your fingers were. If you notice tension in your shoulders, take your hands a bit broader and turn them out a little. Curl your toes under and lift your hips upward and backward. Keep your arms straight as you glance back at your legs. Press down via your index fingers. If you have stiffness in your hamstrings, keep your knees bent. Bend each knee alternately to stretch your hamstrings and calves. Stay in a Downward-Facing Dog for 5 to 10 breaths.

4. Standing Forward Bend (Uttanasana)

With a Twist From Down Dog, move your feet to the front of the mat and come into Standing Forward Bend. If you have stiffness in your hamstrings, keep your knees bent. You can rest your fingertips on a block or the mat, or you can grab opposing elbows and gently sway from side to side. Allow your neck and shoulders to loosen and allow your head to hang heavy. Stay here for 5-10 breaths.

Release your fingertips on the mat or a block, inhale, and rise halfway to extend through your spine in Standing Half Forward Bend. Bend your left knee and stretch your right hand toward the ceiling in a twist. If you have low back pain, place your right hand on your hip instead of extending it toward the ceiling. Lean your head slightly back, and widen across your chest. If it's comfortable, move your eyes toward your right thumb. Stay here for 5 breaths. Switch sides.

5. Squat (Malasana)

From Standing Forward Bend, step your feet an inch or two more apart, and turn your toes slightly out. Bend your knees and drop your sitting bones toward the mat. If your heels aren't on the mat, bring your hands to the floor or blocks in front of you for support, or slide a wrapped blanket or pillow below your heels.

Bring your hands together at your chest or move your hands forward on the mat, round your spine, and let your head dangle to experience a stretch along your back body. Stay in Squat for 5-10 breaths.

6. Pigeon Pose (Eka Pada Rajakapotasana)

Transition from Squat by extending your legs and returning to Standing Forward Bend. Walk your feet back to Down Dog. Bring your left knee near your left wrist and rest your outer left leg on the mat. Bring your left ankle toward your right wrist to a comfortable amount. Lower your right knee and inch it back until you feel a comfortable stretch down the front of your right leg. You might slip a blanket or cushion below your left hip for support. Inhale and elevate your chest, exhale and fold forward, putting your forearms on blocks or the mat and reaching a comfortable position. You can stack your hands and lay your forehead on them.

Relax your jaw and eyes and focus on your breath here, particularly on the exhale. Stay in Pigeon Pose for at least 5 deep breaths and then proceed to Downward-Facing Dog. Pause for several breaths, feeling the difference between your sides. Repeat on your right side.

Variation: If the Pigeon is too severe, you can come onto your back and take Reclining Pigeon. Bend your knees and take your feet flat on the mat approximately hip-distance apart. Bring your left ankle to your right knee to make a figure 4. You can gently push your left thigh or just relax your arms beside your body or rest them on your chest.

7. Bound Angle Pose (Baddha Konasana)

Come to a sitting position on the mat. Draw your feet nearer to each other and move your heels in front of you to produce a diamond shape. If you experience any soreness in the backs of your knees, try placing your feet further away from you or bring a block, folded blanket, or pillow below each knee. Start to lean forward from your hips and allow your spine to round. Lean your chest towards your feet instead of your thighs. Ensure your forward lean is comfortable, whether minimal or more pronounced. Breathe deeply for 5 to 10 counts while in Bound Angle Pose.

8. Head-to-Knee Pose (Janu Sirsasana)

From Bound Angle Pose, raise your hands to your outer thighs and draw your knees together. Stretch your left leg out straight in front of you. Bring your right foot toward your upper inner left thigh like a sitting Tree Pose (Vrksasana). Turn your upper body toward your straight left leg, inhale, and pull your chest up. As you exhale, stretch forward over your left leg. Again, tilt your torso toward your foot rather than your thigh. If you feel any tugging in your lower back, relax yourself back gently. If you feel any tugging behind the knee of your straight leg, wrap a blanket and slip it below that knee. Try to walk your hands toward your front foot or grab a strap or towel around the base of your left foot and hold it with both hands. Stay for 5 to 10 deep breaths in Head-to-Knee Pose. Switch sides.

9. Reclining Twist

Lie on your back, bend your knees, and spread your feet to the width of your mat. Let both legs gradually descend to the left at the same moment like windshield wipers. Place your left hand on your tummy and stretch your right hand out to the side. You can stay here, or, to improve the stretch, place your left foot on your right knee. Stay in a Reclining Twist for 5 to 10 deep breaths. Switch to the second side.

10. Corpse Pose (Savasana)

From Reclining Twist, bring your knees back to center and slide a bolster, rolled blanket, or a pillow underneath your knees. Separate your feet and lay your arms out from your body with your hands toward the ceiling. Close your eyes. If you feel cold, wrap yourself in a blanket. If the lights aren't dim, you can cover your eyes with your arm, the edge of a blanket, or a towel. Intentionally release all of your muscles. Allow yourself to surrender and release the day. Acknowledge and honor your commitment to your practice, appreciating the time you've dedicated to your evening yoga session on the mat. Remain here for at least 5 minutes. You may even take Savasana in bed if you believe you might be able to doze asleep.

Chapter 3

CUSTOMIZING YOUR PRACTICE

Adapting Routines for Different Fitness Levels

How to Adapt Workouts for Different Fitness Levels

When it comes to customizing routines for varied fitness levels, consider the age-old saying: 'Slow and steady wins the race.' Understanding how to adjust your workout program may make all the difference in accomplishing your objectives successfully and safely.

By making smart tweaks and customizations, you can guarantee that your exercises are demanding yet feasible. But what precise tactics should you take to accommodate varied degrees of fitness?

Let's review some fundamental tactics that can help you traverse this trip with confidence and success.

Key Takeaways

Assess fitness level fully for individualized training routines.

Modify intensity based on objectives and current fitness level.

Focus on appropriate forms to prevent injury and enhance outcomes.

Incorporate progression strategies progressively for sustainable improvement.

Assess Current Fitness Level

To begin customizing your routines for different fitness levels, first analyze your present fitness level precisely and honestly. A thorough fitness exam is vital in generating individualized routines that are effective and safe. Consider aspects like strength, endurance, flexibility, and overall health to evaluate where you stand on the fitness continuum. Customized routines are crucial to growth, so create workouts to meet your present skills while still challenging you to improve.

Start by testing your cardiovascular fitness through sports like running, cycling, or swimming to determine your endurance levels. Test your strength using bodyweight workouts or weights to learn your muscular potential. Check your flexibility via stretches to discover where you might need improvement.

Modify Exercise Intensity

Ready to take your workouts to the next level?

Adjusting weights and reps, as well as employing rest periods, may assist in customizing the intensity of your exercises to your fitness level.

Adjusting Weights and Reps

When modifying weights and reps in your exercises, consider your current fitness level and goals to properly adapt the exercise intensity. Customized tweaks and targeted changes are crucial to ensure that your exercises push you correctly.

Start by measuring your strength and endurance capabilities to decide the correct amount of weight to employ. For novices, smaller weights with more reps might help create a foundation. On the other side, if you're more proficient, raising the weight with fewer reps might push you to new limits.

Personalized adaptations and tailored tweaks guarantee that you continue to develop towards your fitness objectives. Remember, the idea is to alter your weights and reps to constantly challenge yourself while keeping perfect technique.

Using Rest Intervals

Adjusting your rest intervals throughout workouts is a clever strategy to vary the intensity of your activities and maximize your training efficacy. By being attentive to your breathing patterns and including active recovery times, you may adapt your rest intervals to match your fitness level and goals.

Shortening rest durations between sets may increase the challenge and keep your heart rate up, great for individuals trying to develop endurance. On the other hand, prolonging rest times allows for more significant recuperation, excellent for strength training aficionados striving for maximal effort on each set.

Focus on Form and Technique

To improve your workout efficacy and minimize injury, emphasize attention to appropriate form and technique throughout your exercise regimen. Proper alignment is vital to ensure the proper muscles are engaged and to reduce pressure on other body components. Pay attention to your body's movement patterns, ensuring smooth and controlled motions to improve muscle engagement and reduce undue stress on joints.

Maintaining appropriate form not only decreases the chance of injury but also helps you target the desired muscle groups more efficiently. For example, during a squat, perfect alignment of your knees over your toes and maintaining your back straight will stimulate your quadriceps and glutes efficiently. This attention to precision in form guarantees that each exercise you undertake produces optimum benefits.

Incorporate Progression Techniques

To further boost your fitness journey and push your body successfully, including progression strategies into your routines is crucial. Progressive overload is a key idea where you steadily raise the intensity, length, or frequency of your exercises to keep pushing your limitations. This might entail increasing greater weight, completing more repetitions, or lowering rest time between sets. As you develop, it's crucial to have regression choices accessible. These changes allow you to ratchet back the challenge as needed, ensuring you retain perfect technique and prevent damage.

In addition to progressive overload, incremental progression is necessary for long-term success. Set tiny, achievable objectives that push you slightly beyond your comfort zone. This strategy helps you stay motivated and measure your progress efficiently. Scaling changes are also helpful tools to tailor workouts to your current fitness level. Whether it's changing the range of motion or employing resistance bands for aid, these changes let you challenge yourself while keeping safe. By using these progression tactics, you'll continue to get stronger and fitter on your fitness quest.

Listen to Your Body

Pay attention to the signals your body is sending during your exercises to ensure you're pushing yourself successfully while keeping safe and injury-free. Mindful movement is crucial to recognizing your body's limits and possibilities. Listen to how your muscles and joints respond to different activities. If you experience any intense pain or discomfort beyond typical muscular weariness, it's crucial to pause and reassess.

Remember, growth is about incremental improvement, not dramatic leaps. By tuning into your body's indications, you may modify your exercises to meet your current fitness level. Body awareness is vital for building a tailored approach to training. Each person is distinct; meaning what is effective for one individual may not be suitable for another.

Take the time to understand what feels appropriate for you, and don't be hesitant to change your workout intensity or program accordingly. Trust yourself to make the proper decisions depending on how your body feels, and you'll set yourself up for success in your fitness journey.

Seek Professional Guidance

Listen to your body's instincts and consider obtaining expert coaching to boost your fitness journey to the next level. Finding a trainer may be a game-changer in helping you personalize your training to your requirements and goals. A trainer may give specialized instruction, support, and accountability, ensuring that you're on the correct road toward attaining your fitness objectives.

Moreover, don't underestimate the potential of internet resources. There's a lot of material accessible online, from workout schedules to instructional videos that may help you learn new exercises, correct your technique, and remain motivated. Many fitness specialists provide virtual coaching sessions, making it easier to obtain expert guidance from the comfort of your home.

Stay Consistent and Patient

You've launched on a road to greater health, and constancy is your best friend. By adhering to your program, you're not only exercising; you're developing a habit that will lead to progress.

Set Realistic Goals

Wondering how to make realistic exercise objectives that keep you motivated while assuring consistent development on your quest to improved health and strength? Here's how you can do it:

- Reflect on Your Why: Understand your motives for wanting to enhance your fitness.
- Start Small: Break down your ultimate aim into smaller, manageable benchmarks.
- Be Specific: Define specific and quantifiable targets to measure your development successfully.
- Celebrate Achievements: Acknowledge and praise yourself for accomplishing each milestone along the road.
- Stay Flexible: Adjust your objectives as required to be challenged and inspired during your fitness journey.

Track Progress Regularly

To stay on track with your fitness journey and observe continual development, it's vital to routinely assess and analyze your progress. Setting specific objectives offers you direction and drive, but measuring your progress is what keeps you accountable and helps you make necessary modifications. Whether it's charting your exercises, assessing your performance, or keeping a journal of how you feel, tracking progress is crucial.

Celebrate Small Victories

As you measure your progress constantly, remember to enjoy the minor triumphs along the path to being consistent and patient in your fitness quest. It's vital to identify and appreciate the progress you accomplish, no matter how modest it may appear.

Here are some ways to help you keep motivated and encouraged:

- Set Achievable Goals: Break down your ultimate aim into smaller, manageable benchmarks.
- Track Your Progress: Keep a journal or use an app to monitor your successes.
- Reward Yourself: Treat yourself when you hit a milestone to keep motivated.
- Share Your Success: Celebrate with friends or family to raise your spirits.
- Stay Positive: Focus on your victories and utilize them as fuel to keep going.

Chapter 4

CHAIR YOGA FOR SPECIFIC NEEDS

Exercises for Improving Balance and Stability

Introduction to balancing exercises

Balance exercises can help you preserve your balance — and confidence — at any age. Balance exercises are especially essential for older persons since they can assist avoid falls and help them preserve their independence. It's a good idea to include balance training along with physical exercise and strength training in your normal activity.

Nearly any exercise that keeps you on your feet and moving, such as walking, will help you preserve good balance. But particular exercises aimed to enhance your balance are important to incorporate into your everyday routine and can assist increase your stability.

For example, balance on one foot when you're standing for some time at home or when you're out and about. Or, rise from a sitting posture without using your hands. Alternatively, attempt walking in a straight line, placing your heel directly in front of your toes, covering a brief distance. You also can attempt tai chi - a sort of movement training that may enhance balance and stability and lessen the incidence of falls.

If you have serious balance issues or an orthopedic disease, obtain your healthcare professional's OK before practicing balancing exercises.

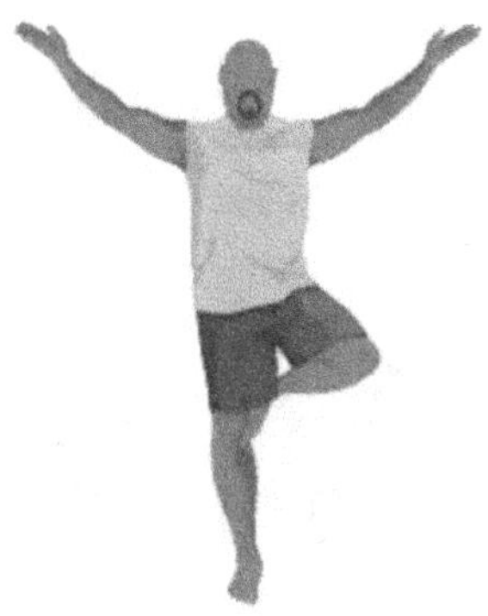

A person stands on one foot with both hands raised in the air.

Weight shifts

When you're ready to undertake balancing exercises, start with weight shifts:

Stand with your feet positioned hip-width apart and your weight evenly distributed between both legs (A).

Shift your weight to your right side, then raise your left foot off the floor (B).

Hold the pose as long as you can preserve good form, up to 30 seconds.

Go back to the initial position and repeat the movement on the opposite side. As your balance improves, increase the amount of repetitions.

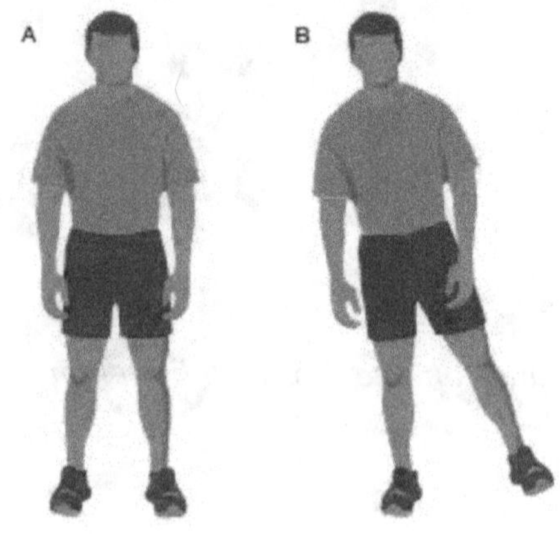

The person conducting weight shifts.

Single-leg balance

Standing on one leg is another frequent balancing exercise:

Stand with your feet positioned hip-width apart, ensuring your weight is evenly distributed between both legs. Place your hands on your hips. Raise your left leg off the floor and bend it backward at the knee (A). If this is too tough at first, you can stand on one leg while holding onto a stable item, such as a piece of heavy furniture or a table.

Hold the pose as long as you can preserve good form, up to 30 seconds.

Return to the initial position and perform the same movement on the opposite side. As your balance improves, increase the amount of repetitions.

For variation, reach out with your foot as far as possible without contacting the floor (B).

For additional effort, balance on one leg while standing on a cushion or other unstable surface.

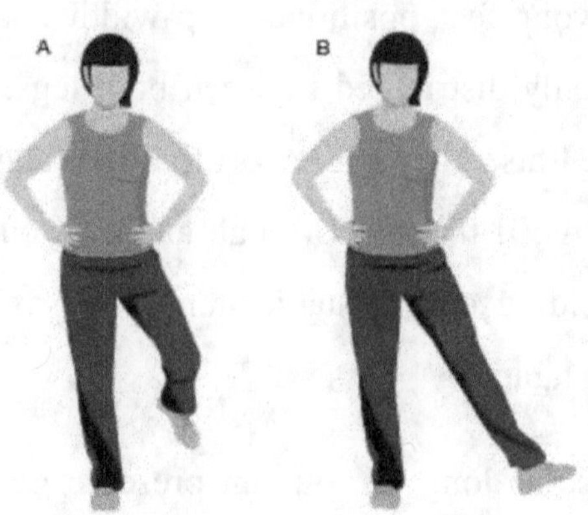

A person practicing single-leg balancing exercises

Bicep curls for balance

Weights may make balancing exercises more hard and also engage core muscles. Try biceps curls with a dumbbell:

Stand with your feet hip-width apart and your weight equally divided over both legs. Hold the dumbbell in your left hand with your palm pointing upward (A). Raise your right leg off the ground and bend it backwards at the knee (B).

Hold the pose as long as you can preserve good form, up to 30 seconds.

Return to the initial position and repeat the exercise on the opposite side. As your balance improves, increase the amount of repetitions.

For further effort, balance on the leg opposite the weight (C) or while standing on a cushion or other unstable surface (D).

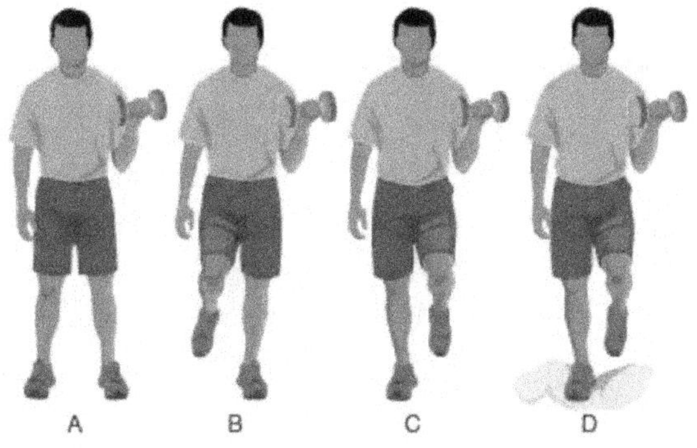

A person practicing biceps curls to enhance balance.

Tai chi for balance

Another activity that might assist improve balance and minimize the risk of falls is tai chi – a sort of movement training.

Look for group classes provided at local fitness facilities or senior centers. Or rent or buy movies or books about tai chi. But bear in mind that it's hard to guarantee you're applying the appropriate strategies while studying the exercises from a book.

Poses for Enhancing Flexibility

Flexibility is one of the important aspects of excellent physical health. Over time, though, your body may lose flexibility due to aging, a sedentary lifestyle, stress, or incorrect posture and movement patterns.

If you're ready to raise your flexibility, consistently practicing yoga, whether in a class or at home, maybe one of the greatest ways Trusted Source to develop mobility in your muscles and joints.

Along with enhancing your flexibility, practicing various yoga postures may also help you improve muscle strength and lessen feelings of tension or worry.

In this post, we'll discuss the benefits of increasing your flexibility and lead you through the greatest yoga poses for building flexibility in your back, hips, core, neck, and shoulders.

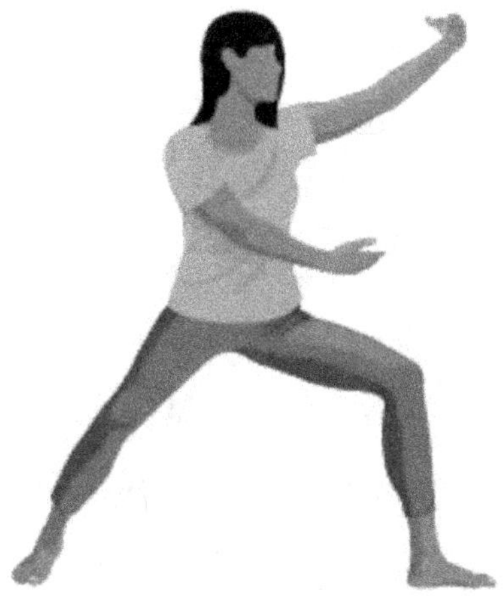

Why is flexibility important?

Increasing your flexibility is helpful for you in many ways. Among the most notable advantages are:

- Greater range of motion. Increased flexibility makes it simpler to move your joints in a normal direction with less effort.

- Less muscular tension. Stretching your muscles can assist relieve tension and tightness, making it simpler to move.

- Better posture. Tight, rigid muscles can contribute to muscular pain and poor posture.

- Less pain. When your muscles aren't stiff, there's typically less tension and strain on particular portions of your body and, as a consequence, less discomfort in your back, neck, and shoulders.

- Lower risk of injury. Enhanced strength and flexibility in your muscles and joints could reduce your susceptibility to injuries.
- Less stress. Releasing tension in your muscles can promote relaxation, potentially reducing your overall stress levels.
- Improved circulation. Better blood flow may help your muscles recover more rapidly after an exercise and also reduce stiffness.

Best yoga positions for enhanced flexibility

If you're interested in trying a yoga class to enhance your flexibility, Hatha, Vinyasa, or Yin styles are all terrific possibilities.

If you're short on time or would like to practice some yoga positions at home, the following poses can be extremely effective for stretching many of your major muscles and enhancing flexibility.

With each posture, go at your own pace. Focus on how the stance feels instead of how it appears. You may perform each posture multiple times, ensuring it feels comfortable and manageable without excessive difficulty.

Poses for back flexibility

1. Intense side stretch (Parsvottanasana)

This forward bend extends your spine, hips, and legs. It also aids your posture, balance, and digestion.

To achieve this pose:

- Stand with your left foot in front looking forward and your right foot back, turning out your toes at a small angle.
- Square both of your hips to face front.
- Place your hands on your hips.
- Bend at your hips to bend your body forward, burying your chin into your chest.
- Lower your hands towards the floor, or rest them on a block.
- Hold this stance for 30 seconds to 1 minute.
- Switch the location of your feet and do the opposite side.

2. Head to knee (Janu Sirsasana)

Suitable for all levels, this position helps increase flexibility in your back, hips, and thighs. It also stimulates blood flow in the lower abdomen and may be a terrific stress reducer.

To execute this pose:

- Sit on the floor or a yoga mat.
- Extend your right leg, and press your left foot onto the inside of your thigh.
- Inhale and lift your arms overhead.
- Exhale and bend at your hips to fold inward toward your extended leg.
- Place your hands on the floor, or hang on to your outstretched leg or foot.
- Hold for 1 to 2 minutes.
- Switch legs and do the opposing side.
- Poses for core flexibility

3. Cat-Cow (Bitilasana Marjaryasana)

The fluidity of this position works great for enhancing mobility and flexibility in your core, neck, shoulders, and spine.

To execute this posture:

- Begin this pose by positioning yourself on all fours, ensuring that your wrists are aligned behind your shoulders and your knees are directly under your hips.
- Keeping your weight spread equally across your body, inhale as you let your belly descend toward the floor. Raise your chest and chin while your tummy goes lower.

- Exhale as you press into your hands to curve your spine up toward the ceiling, tucking your chin into your chest as you do so.
- Continue this exercise for 1 minute.

4. Bow position (Dhanurasana)

This intermediate-level position helps stretch many of the muscles that are engaged when sitting. It can assist enhance flexibility in your core muscles as well as the muscles in your back, chest, glutes, and legs.

Avoid attempting this posture if you have pain or discomfort in your neck, shoulders, or back.

To achieve this pose:

- Lie on your stomach with your arms beside your body.
- Bend your knees and reach back with your hands to hold the outside of your ankles.
- Attempt to raise your shoulders and chest off the ground if possible, but avoid pushing yourself beyond a comfortable limit.
- Keep your head facing ahead while taking long, deep breaths.
- Try to hold for up to 30 seconds, then release.
- Repeat 1 to 2 times.

Poses for hip flexibility

5. Low lunge (Anjaneyasana)

Ideal for all levels, this position helps stretch your spine, expand your hips, and increase muscle power. It may also help treat sciatica.

To execute this pose:

- Position yourself on the floor with your left knee down.
- Bend your right knee and place your right foot flat on the ground in front of you.
- Extend your spine upwards, reaching through the crown of your head.
- Lift your body and arms. Or, you might stretch your arms to the side, perpendicular to the floor.
- Gently press into your right hip.
- Try to keep this posture for at least 30 seconds.
- Switch legs and repeat on the opposing side.

Alignment tip: Prevent your front knee from going past your ankle. Maintain square hips by bringing your rear hip forward.

6. Wide-angle sitting front bend (Upavistha Konasana)

This forward bend can assist open up your hips and lower back while also enhancing flexibility in your hamstrings and calves.

To move further into the posture, you might sit on the edge of a cushion or block to tilt your pelvis forward.

To achieve this pose:

- Sit on the floor with your legs out as far wide as they'll go.
- Extend your arms overhead.
- Hinge at your hips to bend forward, gradually moving your hands closer toward your feet.
- Hold this posture for up to 1 to 2 minutes.

Alignment tip: If your toes point out to the sides, draw your legs in closer. Your toes should face straight up, as though you're slamming the soles of your feet into a wall.

Poses for shoulder and neck flexibility

7. Cow Face Pose (Gomukhasana)

Appropriate for all levels, this position extends your shoulders, chest, and arms.

To execute this pose:

- Position yourself in a comfortable sitting position. Allow your spine to stretch and your chest to open.
- Extend your left arm upward, then bend your elbow so your fingers point down along your back.

- Using your right hand, gently bring your left elbow over to the right, enabling your left hand to slide farther down your spine.
- If it's comfortable, you may try bending your right arm upward along your spine to grasp your left hand.
- Remain in this stance for at least 30 seconds.
- Switch arms and perform the exercise on the opposite side.

8. Plow Pose (Halasana)

This intermediate-level position may assist ease stress in your neck, shoulders, and spine.

If you find it hard for your feet to reach the floor, rest them on the seat of a chair or a stack of pillows. Avoid performing this posture if you have any difficulties with your neck, digestion, or blood pressure.

To execute this pose:

- Lie on your back with your arms beside your body, pushing your hands into the floor.
- Raise your legs straight up to 90 degrees.
- Bring your legs above your head.
- Place your hands on your lower back, positioning your pinky fingers on either side of your spine with your fingers facing upward.

- Hold for 1 to 2 minutes.
- Gradually lower your spine back down to the floor.
- Repeat 1 to 2 times.

Safety Tips

When executing a yoga posture, avoid straining oneself into any position or doing too much too soon. This can raise your chance of harm.

Listen to your body. If a position starts to feel painful or overly unpleasant, release the stance straight away.

You may be able to just hold a position for 10 or 20 seconds at first, and that's just great. As you acquire flexibility, you may work toward holding the positions for longer.

Talk to your doctor or a professional yoga teacher before starting yoga if you:

- Have any injury or pain, including sciatica
- Have high or low blood pressure
- Are menstruating or pregnant have asthma
- Have cardiovascular or respiratory issues
- Have stomach difficulties
- Take any drugs

Chapter 5

PROVEN DELICACIES FOR WEIGHT LOSS

Introduction to Nutritional Support

What characterizes health nutrition?

Embrace a Healthier Lifestyle with Delicious Dishes: Your Complete Guide to Healthy Eating, Nutritious Recipes, and Wellness Journey

Welcome to Delicious Dishes, your go-to site for all things tasty and healthful! At Delicious Dishes, we think that healthy eating is not simply a trend, but a lasting lifestyle choice that can alter your life. Whether you're just starting your health journey or seeking to extend your repertoire of nutritious dishes, we've got you covered.

Healthy Eating: A Lifestyle, Not a Diet

Healthy eating is more than counting calories or following the newest diet craze. It's about making educated decisions that nurture your body and mind. At Delicious Dishes, we highlight the significance of including a range of complete foods in your everyday routine. Think bright fruits and veggies, nutritious grains, lean meats, and healthy fats. These meals are rich in critical nutrients that enhance your energy levels, improve your mood, and promote overall well-being.

Nutritious Recipes: Delicious and Easy to Make

Finding healthful dishes that are both delicious and easy to create may be a struggle. That's when Delicious Dishes comes in. Our handpicked assortment of recipes is meant to make healthy eating pleasant and accessible for everyone. Here are a few of our preferred choices:

1. Quinoa Salad with Avocado and Black Beans

Packed with protein and fiber, this quinoa salad is a terrific dish for lunch or supper. Toss up some cherry tomatoes, corn, and a tangy lime dressing for a blast of flavor.

2. Baked Salmon with Lemon and Dill

This simple yet gorgeous meal is rich in omega-3 fatty acids, which are wonderful for heart health. Serve it with steamed broccoli and brown rice for a balanced supper.

3. Berry and Chia Seed Smoothie Bowl

Start your day with a nutrient-packed smoothie bowl. Blend your favorite fruits with a splash of almond milk, then top with fresh berries, chia seeds, and a sprinkling of granola.

Wellness Journey: Small Steps for Big Changes

Embarking on a wellness path might feel scary, but it doesn't have to be. At Delicious Dishes, we encourage you to take tiny, attainable steps towards healthy living. Here are some pointers to get you started:

1. Plan Your Meals

Plan your meals for the week with careful consideration. This can help you make better choices and avoid the lure of fast food.

2. Stay Hydrated

Drinking adequate water is vital for sustaining good health. Aim for at least eight glasses every day to keep your body hydrated and working effectively.

3. Move Your Body

Incorporate physical activity into your everyday routine. Whether it's a brisk stroll, a yoga session, or a workout at the gym, pick something you love and stay with it.

4. Get Enough Sleep

Quality sleep is vital for general health and well-being. Make sure you're receiving 7-9 hours of sleep each night to allow your body to recover and repair.

At Delicious Dishes, we are devoted to aiding you on your way to a better, happier life. Please browse our website for additional nutritional recipes, healthy eating suggestions, and wellness information. Remember, it's never too late to start your wellness journey. Here's to a healthy you!

Recipes for Breakfast Delicacies

Introduction:

Breakfast is frequently regarded as the most essential meal of the day, and with good reason. A good meal sets the tone for the day, delivering the energy and nutrients required to begin your metabolism and sustain concentration and productivity. In this area, we give a variety of tasty and healthy breakfast dishes meant to complement your chair yoga routine and help your weight reduction objectives.

Recipe 1:

Greek Yogurt Parfait

Ingredients:

- 1 cup of Greek yogurt
- 1/2 cup of fresh berries such as strawberries, blueberries, or raspberries
- 1/4 cup of granola (ideally low-sugar)

- 1 tablespoon of honey - 1 tablespoon of chia seeds

Instructions:

1. In a glass or dish, place half of the Greek yogurt at the bottom.
2. Add a layer of berries, followed by granola.
3. Repeat the layers with the remaining yogurt and berries.
4. Drizzle honey over top and sprinkle with chia seeds.
5. Enjoy immediately for a refreshing and protein-packed start to your day.

Recipe 2:

Spinach and Feta Egg Muffins

Ingredients:

- 6 big eggs
- 1/2 cup of fresh spinach, chopped
- 1/4 cup of crumbled feta cheese - 1/4 cup of chopped tomatoes
- 1/4 cup of chopped bell peppers
- Salt and pepper to taste

Instructions:

1. Preheat your oven to 350°F (175°C) and butter a muffin pan.
2. In a sizable bowl, whisk the eggs until thoroughly combined.

3. Stir in the spinach, feta cheese, tomatoes, and bell peppers.

4. Season with salt and pepper.

5. Pour the egg mixture equally into the muffin tray.

6. Bake for 20-25 minutes, or until the muffins are firm and slightly brown.

7. Allow to cool somewhat before removing from the tin. These may be kept in the refrigerator for up to a week and reheated for a quick breakfast.

Recipe 3:

Oatmeal with Almond Butter and Banana

Ingredients:

- 1/2 cup of rolled oats - 1 cup of water or milk (dairy or non-dairy) 1 banana, sliced
- 1 tablespoon of almond butter
- 1 tablespoon of flaxseeds
- 1 teaspoon of cinnamon

Instructions:

1. In a small saucepan, bring the water or milk to a boil.

2. Add the rolled oats and decrease the heat to a simmer. Simmer for approximately 5 minutes, stirring occasionally.

3. Once the oats are cooked, transfer them to a bowl.

4. Top with banana slices, a dab of almond butter, and a sprinkling of flaxseeds and cinnamon.

5. Serve warm for a substantial and fiber-rich breakfast.

Recipe 4:

Avocado Toast with Poached Egg

Ingredients:

- 1 ripe avocado
- 2 pieces of whole-grain bread - 2 big eggs
- 1 tablespoon of lemon juice
- Salt and pepper to taste
- Optional: red pepper flakes, chives, or cherry tomatoes for garnish

Instructions:

1. Toast the pieces of whole-grain bread to your preferred crispness.

2. While the bread is toasting, put a saucepan of water to a low simmer and poach the eggs (approximately 3-4 minutes for a runny yolk).

3. In a bowl, mash the avocado with lemon juice, salt, and pepper.

4. Spread the mashed avocado equally on the toasted bread.

5. Place a poached egg on top of each piece.

6. Garnish with red pepper flakes, chives, or cherry tomatoes if preferred.

7. Serve immediately for a nutritious and enjoyable breakfast.

Recipe 5:

Berry Smoothie Bowl

Ingredients:

- 1 cup of mixed frozen berries (strawberries, blueberries, raspberries)
- Half a cup of Greek yogurt or plant-based yogurt
- Half a cup of almond milk (or your preferred milk)
- One tablespoon of honey or agave syrup
- A quarter cup of granola
- Fresh berries and mint leaves for garnishing

Instructions:

1. In a blender, mix the frozen berries, Greek yogurt, almond milk, and honey. Blend until smooth.

2. Pour the smoothie into a bowl.

3. Top with granola, fresh berries, and mint leaves.

4. Enjoy with a spoon for a refreshing and antioxidant-rich breakfast choice.

These breakfast dishes are meant to provide you with balanced nourishment, keeping you energized and focused throughout the day. By including these tasty and easy-to-make treats into your morning routine, you may boost the advantages of your chair yoga practice and help your weight reduction journey in a fun way.

Lunch and Dinner Options

Maintaining a balanced diet is a critical component of any successful weight reduction journey, especially for elders and novices. This area presents a choice of tasty and healthy lunch and dinner alternatives that complement your chair yoga exercise, ensuring you acquire the required nutrients while aiding weight reduction.

The Importance of Balanced Meals

Balanced meals are vital for supplying the energy and nutrition needed to sustain your everyday activities and workout regimens. For lunch and supper, focus on a balance of lean meats, nutritious grains, and a variety of veggies. This technique helps to keep you full, control blood sugar levels, and encourage sustained weight reduction.

Nutritious Lunch Recipes

1. Quinoa and Veggie Power Bowl

- Ingredients: Quinoa, chickpeas, cherry tomatoes, cucumber, red bell pepper, feta cheese, lemon-tahini dressing.
- Instructions: Cook quinoa according to package instructions. Combine with chopped veggies and chickpeas. Top with feta cheese and sprinkle with lemon-tahini dressing.

2. Grilled Chicken and Avocado Salad

- Ingredients: Grilled chicken breast, mixed greens, avocado, cherry tomatoes, red onion, balsamic vinaigrette.
- Instructions: Slice cooked chicken breast with avocado. Arrange mixed greens on a platter, and top with chicken, avocado, cherry tomatoes, and red onion. Drizzle with balsamic vinaigrette.

3. Lentil and Spinach Soup

- Ingredients: Green lentils, spinach, carrots, celery, onion, garlic, vegetable broth, thyme.
- Instructions: Sauté chopped onions, carrots, celery, and garlic in a saucepan. Add lentils, vegetable broth, and

thyme. Simmer until lentils are soft. Mix in spinach and simmer until it wilts.

Hearty Dinner Recipes

1. Baked Salmon with Asparagus

- Ingredients: Salmon fillets, asparagus spears, olive oil, lemon slices, garlic, fresh dill.
- Instructions: Preheat oven to 400°F (200°C). Arrange salmon fillets and asparagus on a baking sheet. Drizzle with olive oil, top with lemon slices, chopped garlic, and fresh dill. Cook in the oven for 20 minutes or until the salmon is fully cooked.

2. Turkey and Vegetable Stir-Fry

- Ingredients: Ground turkey, bell peppers, broccoli, snap peas, soy sauce, ginger, garlic.
- Instructions: In a wok or big pan, sauté minced garlic and ginger. Add ground turkey and heat until browned. Add chopped veggies and stir-fry until tender-crisp. Season with soy sauce.

3. Stuffed Bell Peppers

- Ingredients: Bell peppers, lean ground beef or turkey, brown rice, black beans, corn, chopped tomatoes, shredded cheese.

- Instructions: Preheat oven to 375°F (190°C). Trim the tops off the bell peppers and scoop out the seeds. In a bowl, combine cooked brown rice, ground beef, black beans, corn, and chopped tomatoes. Stuff mixture into bell peppers, place in a baking dish, and top with shredded cheese. Bake for 30-35 minutes.

Tips for Preparing Balanced Meals

- Plan Ahead: Prepare ingredients in advance to save time and ensure you have healthy alternatives readily available.

- Portion Control: Be cautious of portion amounts to avoid overeating. Use smaller plates to help regulate portions.

- Hydration: Drink lots of water throughout the day to keep hydrated and help digestion.

Incorporating these lunch and dinner alternatives into your daily routine will help you reach your weight reduction goals while delivering the required nutrients for general health and well-being. By combining these balanced meals with your daily chair yoga practice, you'll be well on your way to a healthier and more active existence.

Healthy Snacks and Smoothies

Healthy snacks and smoothies are crucial components of a balanced diet, especially for those engaged in a workout regimen like chair yoga. These nutrient-dense alternatives give prolonged energy, induce satiety, and help weight reduction by suppressing cravings and limiting overeating. In this part, we'll examine a selection of tasty and easy-to-make snacks and smoothies that are excellent for elders and novices wishing to supplement their chair yoga practice.

The Importance of Healthy Snacks and Smoothies

Healthy snacks and smoothies serve a significant part in sustaining energy levels throughout the day. They can help balance blood sugar, minimize hunger pains, and supply critical nutrients that support general health and well-being. Incorporating them into your routine will increase your workout efforts and assist in healthy weight management.

Nutritious Snack Ideas

1. Greek Yogurt with Fresh Berries

- Ingredients: Greek yogurt, mixed berries (strawberries, blueberries, raspberries), a drizzle of honey
- Benefits: High in protein and antioxidants, this snack is ideal for muscle rehabilitation and improving immunological health.

2. Veggie Sticks with Hummus

- Ingredients: Carrot sticks, cucumber slices, bell pepper strips, homemade or store-bought hummus
- Benefits: Rich in fiber and vitamins, this mix keeps you full and pleased while supporting digestive health.

3. Apple Slices with Almond Butter

- Ingredients: Sliced apples, almond butter
- Benefits: A wonderful source of healthy fats and protein, this snack helps maintain consistent energy levels.

4. Trail Mix

- Ingredients: A blend of nuts (almonds, walnuts), seeds (pumpkin, sunflower), dried fruit (raisins, cranberries), dark chocolate chips

- Benefits: Packed with healthy fats, protein, and antioxidants, trail mix is a fantastic on-the-go snack.

Delicious Smoothie Recipes

1. Green Detox Smoothie

- Ingredients: Spinach, kale, green apple, banana, lemon juice, water, or coconut water
- Benefits: Loaded with vitamins, minerals, and antioxidants, this smoothie assists in detoxifying and improves vitality.

2. Berry Protein Smoothie

- Ingredients: Mixed berries (blueberries, raspberries, strawberries), Greek yogurt, a scoop of protein powder, almond milk
- Benefits: High in protein and antioxidants, this smoothie helps muscle rehabilitation and general health.

3. Tropical Mango Smoothie

- Ingredients: Mango, pineapple, banana, coconut milk, a handful of spinach
- Benefits: Rich in vitamins A and C, this smoothie is refreshing and improves immunological function.

4. Peanut Butter Banana Smoothie

- Ingredients: Banana, peanut butter, Greek yogurt, a touch of honey, almond milk
- Benefits: An excellent dose of protein and healthy fats, this smoothie is perfect for a post-workout snack.

Tips for Making the Perfect Smoothie

1. Balance Your Ingredients: Aim for a combination of fruits, veggies, protein sources, and healthy fats to make a well-rounded smoothie.
2. Use Fresh and Frozen food: Fresh food gives maximum nutrition, while frozen fruits and veggies provide thickness and a delightful chill.
3. Avoid Added Sugars: Opt for natural sweeteners like honey or dates, and be aware of high-sugar products.
4. Experiment with Flavors: Don't be hesitant to test different combinations and ingredients to make your snacks and smoothies intriguing and delectable.

Incorporating these nutritious snacks and smoothies into your daily routine will substantially benefit your weight reduction journey and general health. They give necessary nutrients, assist in maintaining energy levels, and support your chair yoga practice, ensuring you stay fed and energized throughout the day.

Chapter 6

CREATING A HOLISTIC APPROACH

Integrating Chair Yoga with a Balanced Diet

Chair yoga and a balanced diet are complementary components of a holistic wellness strategy, especially for seniors and beginners aiming for weight loss and improved health. This section delves into the importance of combining these two elements, offering practical advice and actionable steps to achieve the best results.

Understanding the Synergy

Combining chair yoga with a balanced diet maximizes the benefits of both practices. Chair yoga enhances physical activity, promoting flexibility, strength, and mental relaxation. A balanced diet provides the necessary nutrients to fuel the body, aid in recovery, and maintain optimal energy levels. Together, they create a sustainable approach to weight loss and overall well-being.

Key Components of a Balanced Diet

1. Macronutrients:

- Proteins: Essential for muscle repair and growth. Include lean meats, fish, beans, and legumes.

- Carbohydrates: Provide energy. Such as whole grains, fruits, and vegetables.
- Fats: Necessary for hormone production and cell health. Choose healthy fats from avocados, nuts, seeds, and olive oil.

2. Micronutrients:

- Vitamins and minerals are essential for a variety of bodily functions. Ensure a diverse intake of fruits, vegetables, nuts, and seeds to cover all essential vitamins and minerals.

3. Hydration:

- Water: Vital for overall health and aids in digestion, circulation, and temperature regulation. Strive to drink at least 8 glasses of water daily.

Integrating Nutrition with Chair Yoga

1. Pre-Yoga Nutrition:

- Timing: Eat a light meal or snack about 1-2 hours before your chair yoga session to provide energy without discomfort.
- Choices: Opt for easily digestible foods such as a smoothie, a piece of fruit with yogurt, or a small portion of oatmeal.

2. Post-Yoga Nutrition:

- Recovery: Focus on replenishing energy stores and aiding muscle recovery with a balanced meal containing proteins, carbs, and healthy fats.
- Examples: A grilled chicken salad with quinoa, a whole-grain wrap with hummus and veggies, or a bowl of Greek yogurt with mixed berries and nuts.

Practical Tips for Integrating Diet and Yoga

1. Meal Planning:

- Consistency: Plan your meals and snacks around your chair yoga schedule to maintain energy levels and support recovery.
- Preparation: Prepare meals in advance to ensure you have healthy options readily available.

2. Mindful Eating:

- Awareness: Practice mindful eating by paying attention to hunger cues, eating slowly, and savoring each bite.
- Portion Control: Be mindful of portion sizes to avoid overeating, especially after yoga sessions.

3. Balanced Meals:

- Include a diverse selection of foods in your diet to ensure you receive a broad spectrum of nutrients.
- Balance: Aim for balanced meals that include a good mix of macronutrients and micronutrients.

Sample Balanced Diet Plan

Breakfast:
- Scrambled eggs with spinach and whole-grain toast.
- Fresh fruit smoothie with protein powder.

Lunch:
- Grilled chicken breast with quinoa and a mixed vegetable salad.
- Lentil soup with a side of whole-grain bread.

Dinner:
- Oven-baked salmon served with brown rice and steamed broccoli.
- Tofu stir-fry with a medley of vegetables and noodles.

Snacks:
- Greek yogurt with honey and walnuts.

- Apple slices with almond butter.

Integrating chair yoga with a balanced diet creates a comprehensive approach to weight loss and overall health. By focusing on nutritious foods and mindful eating practices, you can enhance the benefits of your yoga practice, leading to a healthier, more vibrant life. Remember, consistency is key, and small, sustainable changes will yield the best long-term results.

Mindfulness and Meditation Practices

Incorporating mindfulness and meditation into your chair yoga practice may dramatically boost your overall well-being. These techniques not only help your physical health but also contribute to emotional balance, stress reduction, and mental clarity. This section gives a complete instruction on how to smoothly integrate mindfulness and meditation into your everyday routine, ensuring a holistic approach to wellbeing.

Understanding Mindfulness

Mindfulness is the discipline of being completely present and engaged at the moment, aware of your thoughts, feelings, and sensations without judgment. It entails focusing your attention on the present experience rather than ruminating on the past or worrying about the future. Mindfulness may be cultivated throughout chair yoga sessions and your regular activities.

Benefits of Mindfulness

- Reduces Stress: Mindfulness helps to relax the mind, lessening the physiological impacts of stress.
- Improves Focus: Regular practice strengthens your ability to concentrate and sustain attention.
- Enhances Emotional Regulation: Mindfulness creates a balanced emotional state, helping you control unpleasant emotions more efficiently.
- Boosts Overall Well-being: Practicing mindfulness has been found to increase mental health and general life pleasure.

Techniques for Practicing Mindfulness

1. Mindful Breathing: Focus on your breath as you inhale and exhale. Notice the sensation of the air entering and exiting your body. If your mind wanders, softly bring your focus back to your breath.
2. Body Scan: Sit comfortably in your chair and close your eyes. Slowly direct your focus to different regions of your body,

starting with your toes and progressing up to your head. Notice any feelings, tension, or places of relaxation.

3. Mindful Movement: As you execute chair yoga postures, focus on the flow of your body and the alignment of each pose. Pay attention to how your muscles feel and how your body responds to each stretch and action.

4. Mindful Listening: During your practice, listen to the noises around you without judgment. It may be the sound of your breath, background noise, or even the directions of a guided meditation.

Introduction to Meditation

Meditation is a disciplined practice that includes concentrating the mind to attain a state of calm and heightened awareness. It compliments chair yoga by developing a sense of inner serenity and clarity.

Types of Meditation

- Guided Meditation: Follow along with a recorded or live guide who guides you through a series of visualizations and relaxation methods.

- Mantra Meditation: Repeat a word or phrase (mantra) silently or aloud to focus your thoughts and eliminate distractions.

- Loving-Kindness Meditation: Focus on cultivating sentiments of compassion and love for yourself and others.

- Mindfulness Meditation: Focus on the present moment, monitoring thoughts and feelings without judgment.

How to Incorporate Meditation into Your Chair Yoga Practice

1. Start Small: Begin with only a few minutes of meditation before or after your chair yoga session. Gradually increase the length as you get more comfortable with the exercise.

2. Find a peaceful Space: Choose a peaceful and comfortable area where you may sit undisturbed. Ensure that your chair promotes a comfortable, upright posture.

3. Create an objective: Before commencing your meditation, create a clear objective or goal for your practice. It might be to alleviate tension, boost attention, or simply to relax.

4. Use Guided Meditations: For novices, guided meditations can give structure and assistance. There are numerous resources accessible online or through meditation applications.

5. Be Patient: Meditation is a talent that requires time to perfect. Be patient with yourself and approach the exercise with an open and non-judgmental attitude.

Integrating Mindfulness and Meditation into Daily Life

- Mindful Eating: Pay complete attention to the sensation of eating. Notice the tastes, textures, and fragrances of your meal.
- Mindful Walking: During a stroll, focus on the sensation of your feet touching the ground and the rhythm of your footfall.
- Mindful Communication: Practice active listening and completely engage in discussions without interruptions.

By integrating mindfulness and meditation into your chair yoga practice and daily routine, you may create a deeper feeling of well-being and balance. These activities help you to live more completely in the present moment, supporting a holistic approach to physical and mental health.

Tracking Progress and Staying Motivated

Staying motivated and measuring progress are key components of any fitness program, particularly for elders and beginners engaged in chair yoga for weight reduction. This section contains practical advice and tactics to help you retain excitement, monitor your successes, and overcome hurdles along the road.

1. Setting Realistic and Achievable Goals

Identify Your Starting Point**: Begin by analyzing your current fitness level and weight. This will help you develop realistic and personalized objectives.

- Short-Term and Long-Term Goals: Break down your ultimate ambition into doable stages. Celebrate modest accomplishments to keep motivation strong.
- SMART Goals: Ensure your goals are Specific, Measurable, Achievable, Relevant, and Time-bound. For example, try to lose 5 pounds in the following month via daily chair yoga and a balanced diet.

2. Creating a Progress Tracking System

- Use a Journal or App: Record your daily exercises, noting the time, intensity, and any physical changes. Digital applications can offer extra features like reminders and progress charts.

- Track Physical Changes: Measure your weight, physical measurements, and fitness levels frequently. Note gains in flexibility, balance, and strength.
- Visual Progress: Take before-and-after images to graphically chronicle your transformation. This may be a great incentive.

3. Staying Motivated with a Support System

- Find a Workout Buddy: Partner with a friend or family member to keep each other responsible and motivated. Sharing your journey might make it more pleasant and gratifying.
- Join Online Communities: Engage with individuals who share your aims. Online forums and social media groups may give support, inspiration, and advice.
- Seek Professional Guidance: If feasible, work with a professional chair yoga instructor or a fitness coach who can give individualized recommendations and support.

4. Overcoming Plateaus and Setbacks

- Stay Positive: Accept that development may not always be linear. Plateaus and setbacks are typical components of any fitness regimen.
- Adjust Your Routine: If you encounter a plateau, consider altering your workouts. Introduce new chair yoga postures, increase intensity, or combine other kinds of exercise.
- Reflect and Reassess: Periodically examine your goals and progress. Make modifications as needed to keep on target and continue making progress.

5. Celebrating Your Successes

- Reward Yourself: Indulge in something special as a treat when you achieve a milestone. Choose prizes that correspond with your healthy lifestyle, such as a new yoga mat, a soothing massage, or a favorite nutritious meal.
- Share Your Achievements: Tell your friends and family about your progress. Their good remarks might improve your motivation and confidence.
- Maintain a Positive Mindset: Focus on the benefits you've received, such as more energy, enhanced flexibility, and better general health. Celebrate your devotion and dedication.

Tracking your progress and remaining motivated are key to attaining permanent effects with chair yoga for weight reduction. By setting reasonable objectives, building a support system, and having a positive mentality, you may manage hurdles and enjoy your triumphs on this wonderful journey.

Chapter 7

SUCCESS STORIES AND TESTIMONIALS

Embracing Wellness: Personal Stories of Transformation

In this chapter, we dig into inspirational accounts from individuals who have embraced chair yoga as a transforming practice in their lives. These anecdotes show the many advantages of chair yoga beyond physical fitness, including enhanced mental clarity, emotional balance, and general well-being.

Jane's Journey to Strength

Jane, a former teacher, discusses how chair yoga helped her rebuild strength and flexibility following hip surgery. Through constant exercise, she not only restored mobility but also discovered a renewed feeling of confidence and tranquility.

Mark's Mental Clarity

Mark, a busy professional, recounts how chair yoga became his anchor in a frantic schedule. The mindfulness skills taught in class helped him manage stress and keep focus throughout the day.

Maria's Community Connection

Maria, a senior living community member, recounts the sense of community developed by chairing yoga courses. These sessions not only helped her physical condition but also developed lifelong friendships and a support network.

Enhancing Quality of Life: Practical Insights and Lessons Learned

In addition to personal anecdotes, this part contains practical ideas and lessons learned from chair yoga practitioners of all backgrounds. These insights include ideas on adjusting postures for particular needs, incorporating yoga into daily routines, and facing hurdles with perseverance and drive.

- Tips for Beginners: Practical advice from beginners who overcame first hesitations and discovered the advantages of chair yoga.
- Long-term Benefits: Testimonials from long-time practitioners who relate how chair yoga has helped their general quality of life, from improved posture to better sleep and reduced joint discomfort.
- Instructor Perspectives: Perspectives from certified chair yoga teachers on the transforming nature of the practice and its beneficial influence on their students' lives.

This chapter intends to inspire readers with real-life examples that highlight the enormous influence of chair yoga on physical health, emotional well-being, and community connection.

Tips and Advice from Experienced Instructors

Incorporating chair yoga into your daily practice may be enormously beneficial for both physical and emotional well-being. Here are important ideas and insights from experienced instructors to boost your chair yoga practice:

1. Start Slow and Listen to Your Body

Begin with simple stretches and exercises that feel comfortable. Respect your body's limitations and progressively increase intensity over time.

2. Focus on Breathing

Deep, thoughtful breathing is crucial to chair yoga. Coordinate your breath with each action to boost relaxation and promote better oxygenation.

3. Use Props for Support

Utilize cushions, blocks, or belts to alter positions and offer support where needed. Props can assist in maintaining appropriate alignment and reduce strain.

4. Stay Consistent

Regular practice produces the best outcomes. Aim for daily or several times a week to receive the full advantages of chair yoga, including greater flexibility, strength, and mental clarity.

5. Explore Different Positions

Experiment with a range of chair yoga positions to address different muscle groups and areas of stress. This variability keeps your practice exciting and successful.

6. Awareness and Relaxation

Incorporate periods of awareness and relaxation into your practice. Focus on the present moment, release stress, and build a sense of tranquility.

7. Modify positions for Comfort

Adjust positions to fit your comfort level and physical condition. Honor your body's demands and make adaptations as required to minimize harm and optimize benefits.

8. Combine with Healthy Eating Habits

Pair chair yoga with a balanced diet rich in nutrients. This holistic approach improves weight control, boosts energy levels, and promotes overall vitality.

9. Seek Guidance from Qualified Teachers

Attend sessions conducted by trained chair yoga teachers or check with healthcare specialists before starting a new workout program, especially if you have specific health issues.

10. Appreciate Your Progress

Acknowledge and appreciate each milestone in your chair yoga journey. Whether it's enhanced flexibility, lower stress, or better posture, every success is a testimonial to your commitment to well-being.

By integrating these principles into your chair yoga practice, you may build a lasting and gratifying health habit that feeds both body and mind.

9 798332 458606